Rosacea Reducing Smoothies

Berry Of The Sea

½ cup fresh blackberries
½ cup fresh raspberries
1-cup seaweed (nori or kelp)
10 ounces filtered water
3-cup ice

- Chef's notes for all smoothies follow the following procedure.
- Blend in blender or smoothie maker and add water last until you reach your desired consistency.

Black Melon Sweetie

1-cup fresh blackberries
1-cup fresh diced seedless watermelon
1-cup seaweed (nori or kelp)
1-tblsp. Chopped fresh mint
10 ounces filtered water
3-cup ice

The Athletic Cherry

1-cup fresh-pitted cherries
1-cup pomegranate juice
1 scoop vanilla protein powder (optional)
1-tblsp. Fresh chopped mint
10 ounces filtered water
3-cup ice

Sweet cherry Pie

1-cup fresh cherries pitted
1/2 –cup fresh blueberries
1-cup orange juice

1-tblsp. Fresh chopped mint
10 ounces filtered water
3-cup ice

Very Berry Cobbler

1-cup fresh or frozen blueberries
1-cup fresh or frozen blackberries
½-cup almond milk
1 1/2-tblsp. Flaxseed meal
1-tsp. lemon juice and zest from half rind
1-tblsp. Fresh chopped mint
10 ounces filtered water
Pinch of nutmeg
3-cup ice

Twisted Pumpkin

½-cup pumpkin puree
1-cup orange juice
½-cup almond milk
1 ½-tblsp. Flaxseed meal
3-cups ice cubes
1-tblsp fresh chopped thyme
Pinch of nutmeg

The Crazy Uncle

2-cups honeydew
1-cup blackberries
½- cup pomegranate juice
½-serving vanilla protein powder (optional)
1-tblsp. Flaxseed meal
1-tblsp. Fresh chopped mint
½-tblsp. Fresh thyme
10 ounces filtered water
3-cups ice cubes

What The Tofu

1-cup fresh or frozen cherries
1-cup fresh melon (honeydew or cantaloupe)
1/2 –cup pomegranate juice
1-tblsp. Fresh chopped mint
3 ounces silken tofu (light or Mori-nu)
3-cups ice cubes
10 ounces filtered water

The Strawberry Vixen

1- cup fresh strawberries
½-cup fresh-pitted cherries
1-cup orange juice
2 ounces silken tofu (light or Mori-nu)
1-tblsp. Fresh chopped mint
3-cups ice cubes
10 ounces filtered water

The Simpleton

2-cup fresh mixed berries (your choice)
1-cup orange juice or pomegranate
1-tblsp fresh mint or thyme
3-cups ice cubes
5 ounces filtered water

Tasty Rosacean Apps & Sides

Smoked Trout with Toasted Nori Mayo

4 ounces skinned smoked trout fillets, flaked with fork
¼ cup celery minced
¼ cup carrots cleaned and minced
1-tblsp. Shallots minced
1-tblsp. Lemon juice and zest of ½ lemon
2-tblsp. Limejuice and zest of ½ lime

1-tblsp. Fresh dill
1/4 cup Canola oil

Mix all ingredients in mixing bowl and set aside in fridge to cool.

For the Nori Mayo-

3-5 toasted nori sheets, chopped
1-cup mayonnaise
2-tblsp. Fresh lemon juice
1-tblsp. Fresh limejuice
Zest from half lemon and lime

Finely grind nori in blender or spice mill. Mix nori with mayo, lemon and limejuice, add zest and season with salt if you would like to taste. Mix all thoroughly and cover and chill. This can be made up to 3 days ahead.
- I like to combine this with salad wraps or top on my favorite selection of crackers or whole grain pita.
- Explore this recipe and get creative, be your own chef!

Turkey and kale Stuffed Sweet Potatoes

4 sweet potatoes
½ bunch kale washed and stems removed (rough chopped)
¼ pound ground turkey (cooked and drained)
¼ cup hazelnuts chopped (if you have allergy to these use walnuts)
1 clove garlic minced
1-tblsp. Fresh thyme (pulled from stem)
1-tblsp. Fresh cilantro (chopped)
2-tblsp-canola oil

Preheat oven to 450 degrees
Wash and pierce sweets with fork or paring knife carefully
Wrap in foil and bake on center rack for 55-65 minutes until tender to push on.

While those are cooking cook and crumble turkey with kale and strain and place in mixing bowl. Add fresh herbs, oil, hazelnuts to mixture and fold thoroughly with hands or mixing spoon. Set aside. Unwrap sweets and cut slit down center of each and open carefully by sides using hands, scoop out small amount of each and add to turkey/kale mix. Fold once more and scoop mixture into each potato and place on baking dish or sheet pan. Place back in oven for 10 minutes. Remove from oven let cool to room temp. And enjoy!

Flaxseed Crusted Tofu Bites

1 block tofu (extra-firm and pressed)
1 large egg
¾ cup flaxseed meal
1-tblsp. Fresh (chopped) or dry tarragon
Canola oil for cooking

Press and cut tofu into 1-inch cubes. Combine flaxseed and tarragon in small bowl. Add egg and mix with fork in separate bowl. Heat cast iron skillet or your use your favorite sauté pan and add canola oil over medium heat. Once oil is hot dip tofu cubes in egg bath then dredge in flaxseed mix on all sides coating evenly. Sear in pan until brown all sides about 4-6 minutes. Remove from heat and place on paper towel to dry off. Enjoy!
-   I like to serve these with the toasted nori mayo on following page or use your favorite sauce like sweet and sour. Just remember any spicy sauce or vinegar based will aggravate our symptoms of Rosacea.

Summertime Melon Sliders

1 seedless watermelon cut into ½ disks
2 cucumbers peeled and sliced into ¼ inch disks
½ cup fresh chopped mint
1-pound feta cheese crumbled
Fresh all natural honey for drizzling

Cut both melon and cucumber into disks. Find a cup in your kitchen that is same circumference as your cucumber when sliced. Cut equal sizes from watermelon creating little disks that match your cucumber. Start building your sliders by placing one piece melon on prep surface or plate and top with sprinkle of feta, pinch of mint and drizzle of honey. Top with cucumber slice and again pinch of feta, mint and drizzle of honey. Repeat this 2 more times to build up your slider. Or build it how high you would like (you can always use little skewers and make kabobs as well), these can even be grilled like that for 1 minute a side on medium heat. These can be made up to 3 days ahead and stored in fridge wrapped or covered. Enjoy!

Blackberry and Chicken Bruschetta

½ pound fresh cleaned blackberries (chopped)
½ pound boneless skinless chicken cooked and chopped
¼ cup pomegranate juice
3-tblsp. Fresh chopped basil
2-tblsp. Fresh chopped mint
1-tbslp. Fresh minced garlic (or fresh from jar)
1-tbslp. Canola oil
1- whole grain baguette or your favorite loaf like Focaccia or Ciabatta

Combine first 7 ingredients in mixing bowl and blend well to let flavors build; this is the best when made the day ahead and sits over night in fridge.

Preheat oven to 400 degrees. Cut your bread of choice on flat surface and diagonal to length of bread. Lay your bread on baking sheet or foil and top with chicken blackberry mixture. Bake for 7-10 minutes until bread becomes golden on top. Remove from oven let cool to room temp. And Enjoy!
-   Remember if you drizzle this with balsamic or any other vinegar afterwards you will be subject to facial flushing and flare-ups in your skin.

Flaxseed Zucchini Bites

3 ½ cups sliced and washed zucchini
1 ¼ cup flaxseed meal
¼ cup red onion or Spanish diced
3 large eggs
¼ cup canola oil
1-tblsp. Fresh thyme (pulled from stem)
1-tbslp. Fresh cilantro chopped

Preheat oven to 350 degrees. Mix all ingredients in large bowl and combine thoroughly. Grease an 8x8 or 9x13 baking dish lightly with canola oil and spread in mixture. Bake at 350 for 25-30 minutes until bubbly and top becomes slightly golden brown. Pull from oven and let cool to room temp. Cut into desired pieces (squares) or whatever shape you like and serve at room temp. –Enjoy!

Marinated Beets and Potatoes

4 beets, roasted
3-tbslp. Canola oil
1-pound Yukon gold or red potatoes (red our my favorite way to make this)
1 shallot diced and minced
3-tblsp. Fresh dill
2-tblsp. Fresh thyme

Preheat oven to 400 degrees and wash then wrap beets in foil and roast directly on shelf in middle of oven for 50 minutes. On the top shelf or if there is room same shelf wash and roast the potatoes in shallow baking dish for 40 -50 minutes. When the beets and potatoes are finished and cooled to room temp cube both to desired size and toss into mixing bowl with rest of herbs, oil and shallot. Toss to coat evenly and chill for one hour. -Enjoy!

-   This recipe is very good served at room temp after it is prepared or toss over a bowl of your favorite greens like watercress or escarole. Remember if you use spinach it is high in histamine and is a trigger for your rosacea.

Pomegranate and Blueberry Bruschetta

1 French baguette or whole grain loaf of choice
¼ cup canola oil
1-cup pomegranate aerials (the seeds from the fruit itself)
½ lemon Zested and juiced
½ lime Zested juiced
1½-cup fresh or frozen blueberries
3-tblsp. Fresh mint chopped

Slice bread into pieces big enough to hold in hand and top with berry mixture. Toss all fresh ingredients into mixing bowl and fold to meld the flavors. (This can be done 2 days ahead of time for better results) preheat oven to 400 degrees and top each bread piece with berry mixture. Bake at 400 for 6-8 minutes until bubbly on top and slightly golden. Remove from heat and let cool to room temp-Enjoy!

Cherry and Pumpkin Walnut Bites

½ cup pumpkin puree
2 ounces goat cheese (room temperature)
30 walnut halves (if you have allergy to walnut use full pecan pieces)
¼ cup pitted and chopped cherries
2-tblsp. Fresh chopped cilantro

Combine pumpkin puree and goat cheese in mixing bowl and fold until well incorporated. Set aside. Place walnut halves or almonds on serving dish and top each piece with pumpkin mixture. Place piece of cherry on top each one and finish with small pinch of fresh chopped cilantro (you can even use mint if you want it more fragrant)-Enjoy!

Mixed Berry Caprese Kabobs

2-cup fresh blueberries washed
2-cup fresh blackberries washed
2-cup fresh cherries pitted and washed
1 pack fresh mint washed and patted dry
1 package 6oz. fresh mozzarella pearls
12-18 bamboo skewers (6inch)

Tear each mint leaf in half with you finger carefully. Layer on the bamboo stick one berry of choice then pearl of cheese then piece of mint. Continue to do this and alternate berry so they become very vibrant and colorful. When you are done place in dish and refrigerate until ready to serve. This can be made up to a day ahead and can be served at room temp. These also make great edible decorations in a pitcher of sangria. (Careful not to bite the skewer) –Enjoy!

Facial Flushing Friendly Soups and Salads

Tofutastic Salad

1-pound firm or extra firm tofu (pressed)
3-4 shallots diced and minced
3 stalks celery (diced)
2 carrots peeled and diced
½-cup fresh pitted and chopped cherries
1-¼ cup walnuts (if you have allergy use almond or hazelnut)
1 head Bibb lettuce or head of Romaine

Cut tofu into ½ inch cubes. In mixing bowl, add remaining ingredients, except lettuce and combine well, add tofu and fold in gently. Plate over favorite lettuce chopped or scoop into Bibb lettuce bowl to make a nice presentation. – Enjoy!
- For the dressing, I will discuss sever dressings to make that are non-vinegar based and Rosacea friendly. Make a few and find what works best for you, these can be used on any of the salads here.

Creamy Herb Dressing

¾-cup canola oil
¼ cup fresh mint minced and chopped
¼ cup fresh thyme chopped
¼ cup fresh parsley minced
2- shallots minced
2-tbslp. Parmesan cheese (grated)
2-tblsp. Fresh yogurt (plain)

Combine all ingredients and mix well. Place in storage container to be refrigerated and store for up to one week.

Twisted cheery dressing

¾ cup canola oil
½ cup chopped walnuts or almonds if you have allergy
2 shallots minced
2 cups fresh chopped pitted cherries

1-tblsp. Fresh chopped cilantro
1-tblsp. Fresh chopped mint
1 lemon juiced and zested

Combine all ingredients and blend well. Place in storage container to be refrigerated and store for up to one week.

Plain Jane

¾ cup canola oil
1-tblsp. Fresh herbs chopped of your choice. (Thyme, cilantro, basil)
2 shallots chopped and minced
1 lemon juiced and zested
1 lime juiced and zested
2-tbslp. Plain yogurt

Combine all ingredients and blend well. Place in storage container to be refrigerated and store for up to one week.

Southern Ranch Delight

2-tblsp. Shallots minced
1-tsp garlic chopped fresh or dry
1-tblsp. Fresh chopped parsley or dry
1-tblsp. fresh dill chopped or dry
½ cup buttermilk
½ cup mayonnaise

Combine all ingredients and blend well. Place in storage container to be refrigerated and store for up to one week.

The Serious Walnut

2 cloves garlic smashed and minced
1-tblsp. Fresh chopped thyme
1-tblsp. Tarragon dried
1-tblsp. Fresh parsley chopped or dry is fine
2-½ cups mayonnaise
½ cup buttermilk

1 cup chopped walnuts (If you have allergy use almonds or hazelnuts for great results)

Combine all ingredients in blender and blend until well incorporated. Remove from blender and pour into airtight container for storage in refrigerator. This can be stored for up to two weeks.

The Mighty Grain Salad

2 cups of quinoa cooked and chilled
¼ bunch scallions washed and chopped
1-tblsp. Raw chopped almonds
2-tblsp. Flaxseeds ground
1 lemon juiced and zested
1-tblsp. Fresh chopped garlic
1-cup raisins slightly chopped
¼ cup canola oil

Cook quinoa as directed on box, chill and set aside. Sauté in 1-tblsp. Canola oil, onions, garlic, and almonds until garlic becomes fragrant. Add flaxseed, lemon juice and zest, and raisins and toss to coat evenly. Remove from heat and stir mixture into the quinoa. Drizzle canola oil in to loosen it up and you combine the ingredients well. Chill and serve over your favorite greens like watercress or kale. Remembering spinach is high in histamine and will aggravate your symptoms. This can be made a day ahead of time and can store for up to 5 days.
   -   A little shaved Parmesan on top does wonders for this already excellent super salad.

Very-Berry Salad

½ seedless watermelon cleaned and cut into 1 inch cubes
1-cup fresh blueberries
1-cup fresh blackberries (optional)
½ cup fresh chopped mint
¼ cup fresh chopped basil
1 lemon juiced and zested

1 lime juiced and zested
2-tbslp. Flaxseed (optional)

Combine all ingredients in large mixing bowl and toss evenly to coat well. Remove from bowl and place in container to refrigerate. This can be made up to 2 days a head and store for u to one week.-Enjoy!
- This is excellent served on a nice hot day to help cool our faces, or even added to a smoothie when you have only a few servings left.

Watercress and Blackberry Salad

1 Package watercress washed and rough chopped
4-tblsp. Pumpkin seeds
2-tblsp. Flaxseed
1 small red onion peeled and cut thinly
½ cup walnuts chopped (almonds if your allergic)
2-cup fresh washed blackberries
1-tblsp. Fresh chopped mint

Combine all ingredients in large mixing bowl and toss to incorporate. This can be made a few hours ahead and store for up to one day. - Some fresh goat cheese crumbled on top of salad goes along way and improves the flavor of the berries. -Enjoy!

Cucumbers and Cherries over Watercress

1 English seedless cucumber washed peeled and diced
2 cups watercress leaves washed and rinsed
1 ½ cups washed fresh pitted and chopped cherries
2-tblsp. Fresh dill
2-tblsp. Fresh mint chopped
2-tblsp. Canola oil

Combine all ingredients and toss to coast evenly. This can be made the morning of a dinner or party and can store for up to 2 days in the refrigerator. -Enjoy
- For added touch top salad with some crumbled feta cheese.

Smoked Fish Chowder with Leeks

2-tblsp. Canola oil

3-tblsp. Fresh chopped garlic (dry is fine)

2 cups chopped leeks (white part only)

½ cup diced and peeled red potatoes

12 cups filtered water

8-oz. -smoked trout chopped

8-oz smoked salmon chopped

4-oz. Cod filet chopped

½ cup heavy cream

3-tblsp. Fresh chopped thyme

2-tblsp. Fresh chopped tarragon (dry is fine)

First start by adding oil and leeks and garlic to large soup pot or saucepot. Cook until garlic become fragrant stirring with wooden spoon or one of choice. Add potatoes, water, and cream and bring to simmer. Add fish and herbs and reduce heat to low and simmer this for 1-½ hours. Stirring occasionally. Once this starts to thicken up and smell fragrant remove from stove and let sit to cool to room temp. Serve soup in bowls with pinch of fresh thyme and tarragon and top with sprinkle of sea salt. – Enjoy!

- For an added touch and presentation serve this in bread bowls of your choice.

<u>Zucchini and Squash Bisque</u>

1 ½ cups cooked and cubed butternut squash

1 ½ cups cooked and cubed zucchini

Half of Spanish onion diced or 6 shallots minced

3 stalks celery diced

2 carrots cleaned and diced

2 clove garlic minced or 1-tblsp. Dry

1-tblsp. Fresh thyme

5 Sage leaves chopped and minced

Pinch of nutmeg

10 cups filtered water

2 cups vegetable stock (I use store bought)

½ cup heavy cream

In a large stockpot heat canola oil, garlic, celery, and carrot. Stir until vegetables are tender. Add herbs, squash, and zucchini and stir well to incorporate. Add broth, water and cream to pot and bring to low simmer. Cook this for about 40 minutes and remove from heat and let cool to room temp or use ice wand and chill quicker. Using a ladle scoop this mixture into blender or food processor and carefully blend until smooth. Pour all remaining ingredients into saucepot and heat to serve or serve at room temp. This dish can also be served in a bread bowl for fantastic results. Enjoy!

Berry Grateful Soup

3 cups fresh-pitted tart cherries
2 cups fresh blackberries
2 cups honey dew melon peeled and diced
8 cups filtered water
1-tblsp. Fresh chopped mint
1-tsp. fresh chopped cilantro

In a large saucepan bring berries, herbs, and water to boil. Reduce heat to simmer and let cook for about 15 minutes. Add water if you think its to thick or to your desired consistency. Remove from heat and let cool to room temperature. - Store this soup in airtight container. This can be stored for up to 3 days in fridge. -Enjoy!
-    Chefs tip: place dollop of plain yogurt on top of soup with pinch of fresh chopped mint for added presentation and taste.

White Corn Bisque with Tofu Croutons

3-tblsp. Canola oil
4 stalks celery-diced
1 carrot peeled and diced
1-tblsp. Fresh thyme
1-tsp. Cilantro (dry is fine)
5 cups white corn kernels
10 cups vegetable stock
2 cups filtered water
1-cup heavy cream

1 package firm pressed tofu
3-tblsp. Flax seed

Add celery, carrot, and garlic to sauce pot and cook on medium heat in canola oil. Cook until they become soft and then add thyme and cilantro. Cook for another 2-3 minutes. Add corn and cook for another 3 minutes stirring. Add vegetable stock, filtered water and heavy cream and simmer for about 15-20 minutes more until this is very fragrant and reduces just a bit. Reduce heat and cook another 10 minutes. Remove from heat and set aside to cool. You can either puree this with an immersion blender and finish now or let cool or add a ladle at a time to a blender and process until smooth. Set aside and start on croutons. For the croutons cut tofu into small ¼ inch cubes and place in baking dish with flaxseed. Toss to coat all pieces evenly. Heat sauté pan with canola oil and sear each piece of tofu on all sides until golden brown and producing a nice sear. Remove and place on paper towel to let dry off and cool. Ladle the soup into serving bowl and garnish with tofu croutons. –Enjoy!

Chicken and Green Been Soup with Cherries

1-pound boneless chicken breast cleaned cooked and cubed
½ pound fresh cleaned and chopped green beans
2-tblsp. Fresh chopped garlic (dry is fine)
2-tblsp. Fresh chopped cilantro
2-tblsp. Fresh chopped thyme
2-tblsp. Fresh minced sage
2 stalks celery minced
2 carrots cleaned and chopped
2 cups red potatoes cleaned and chopped
½ yellow onion or 5 shallots minced
1 cup pitted and chopped cherries
5 cups vegetable stock and 10 cups filtered water
Canola oil for cooking

Preheat oven to 325 and bake chicken in baking dish for 25-30 minutes until cooked through, remove cool and chop into cubes. In large stockpot add 1-tblsp. Oil, garlic, celery, carrot, onion and potato. Cook for 4 minutes and stir. Add stock, chicken, green beans, water, and herbs to pot and bring to boil. Cook for 10 minutes and reduce heat to simmer and cook for 35 minutes until soup reduces by ¼. Add cherries stir and Remove from heat and let cool to room temperature. Boil your favorite noodles and serve. (I like to use whole grain small ziti noodles)-Enjoy!

Rosacean Sandwiches

Tart Cherry Tuna Salad Wraps

8 ounces albacore tuna canned in water and drained
¼ cup tart pitted cherries chopped
2-tblsp. Walnuts chopped (pecans if you have allergy)
2-tblsp. Canola oil
1 lemon juiced and zested
1 lime juice and zested
I head Bibb lettuce or your favorite lettuce to make wraps like leaf or romaine, I just prefer Bibb. (Looks nicer)

Combine all ingredients except lettuce in mixing bowl and fold ingredients together to incorporate well. This can be made a day ahead of time and will produce more flavor when done this way as it sits over night. Scoop your tuna salad into your favorite lettuce wrap and serve. -Enjoy!
-   This can also be placed on fresh whole multi grain bread or ciabatta for great flavor.

Crispy Tofu w/ Mint Peanut Sauce and Vegetable Slaw

1 loaf multigrain bread or focaccia sliced (pitas will work too)
1 package extra firm tofu, pressed for 25 minutes
2-tblsp. Canola oil

For the sauce:
½ cup Coconut milk or water is fine
1-tblsp. Walnuts chopped (almond or pecan is fine too if you have allergy)
5-tblsp. Peanut butter (creamy)
1 lime juiced and zested

For the Slaw:

2 carrots peeled and shredded or sliced very thin, (I like to use a potato peeler to make long thin ribbons)
3-4 scallions diced small
2-tbslp. Fresh chopped cilantro
1-tblsp. Fresh chopped mint
1 lemon juiced and zested
2-tblsp. Canola oil

Cut tofu into 8 slices, cutting into triangle and crosswise. Heat oil in large skillet or pan and cook about 4 minutes a side over medium heat until golden and crispy. Remove from heat and place on plate lined with paper towels to let dry and cool.
Meanwhile make the sauce by adding all ingredients to small bowl and whisking together evenly and place in fridge to cool. Now for the slaw again add all ingredients to a larger mixing bowl and fold well into each other and place in fridge to cool. The sauce and slaw can be made up to 2 days ahead of time and can store for up to 5 days in fridge.

Arrange your tofu on your bread of choice and top with sauce and large spoon full of slaw and serve. -Enjoy!

Smoked Salmon w/ Red Onion and Blackberry Relish

8 ounces thinly sliced smoked salmon
10 slices whole grain multi grain bread or you can use leaf lettuce and make this into wraps

For the relish:
1 ½ cups chopped and diced red onion
¼ cup washed and chopped blackberries
2-tblsp. Chopped cilantro
2-tblsp. Drained capers (optional)
1-tblsp. Fresh dill
½ lime juiced and zested
½ lemon juiced and zested

Mix all ingredients for the relish in small bowl and fold well into each other and chill. This can be made a day ahead of time. Take the salmon that is sliced and layer on your piece of bread and top with your red onion relish. If you decide to use lettuce and make wraps scoop relish into wraps and place 2-4 pieces of salmon on top and serve. -Enjoy!

Flaxseed Crusted Cod with Cilantro Aioli

4-tblsp. Flaxseed
2-tbslp. Canola oil
4 4-6 ounce cod filets from market
4 multi grain hoagie buns or 8 slices of whole grain bread of your choice

½ cup mayonnaise
½ lemon juiced and zested
½ lime juiced and zested
2-tbslp. Fresh chopped cilantro
1-tsp. fresh chopped mint

Pre-heat oven to 400 degrees. Combine the mayonnaise, lemon, lime, and herbs in small bowl and mix well. Set in fridge to chill until later. Place you flax seed in small bowl and dredge each piece of fish in and rub on all sides until well coated. Heat oil in skillet on medium heat. When the skillet heats up sear your fish for 4-6 minutes on each side. Once you have cooked each fish remove from heat and place skillet in oven to finish the fish. Finish fish in oven for 10 minutes. Remove from heat and let sit and cool to room temp. Assemble your sandwiches on plates by spreading your cilantro aioli on the bun or bread and top with your fish and serve. -Enjoy!
   - You can also use leaf lettuce or Bibb to make healthy cod wraps.

Sweet Potato Quinoa Burger

Ingredients
2 medium baked sweet potatoes, removed skins and mashed with fork
2 cups cooked quinoa
4 shallots diced
2 cloves garlic mashed and minced
2-tblsp. Fresh thyme
1-tblsp. Fresh cilantro chopped
2-tblsp. Canola oil
1-tblsp. Canola oil for cooking

Prepare your quinoa following package instructions. Preheat oven to 400 degrees and wash and pierce sweet potatoes with fork or paring knife and wrap in foil and bake for 45-55 minutes until tender, remove and let cool to room temp. Remove skins from potatoes and mash with fork and place in large mixing bowl, add quinoa and set aside. In a sauté pan cook onions, canola oil, garlic and half of the thyme over medium heat 3-4 minutes. Remove from heat and add mixture to your bowl of mashed potato and quinoa and mix well to incorporate all flavors. Add last tablespoon of fresh thyme and mix once more. Form mixture into 4-ounce balls (abut the size of large meatball), flatten into patty and set aside on plate for cooking. Heat sauté pan or skillet is better and cook in 1-tblsp canola oil about 2-3 minutes aside until they get golden brown and a little crispy. Make as many as your serving to family or guests and refrigerate the rest of mixture for 3-5 days. - Enjoy!

Cherry Crab Cake Sand with Jicama-Mint Slaw

2-tblsp. Canola oil
4 shallots diced and minced
1-cup fresh whole grain bread crumbs (I like to rip apart my own fresh bread and make my own)
3-tblsp. Fresh chopped cilantro
1-cup fresh pitted chopped cherries
3-egg whites (I save the yolks for the kids French toast)
1 lemon zested and juiced
1 lime zested and juiced
1-lb. fresh Dungeness crab meat or your favorite crabmeat form the market

For the slaw
- Combine 2 cups fresh peeled, julienned jicama, and 2-tblsp. Fresh chopped mint, 1 lemon and 1 lime juiced and zested and combine in bowl. Set aside in fridge to chill.

In a large mixing bowl mix all ingredients except for canola oil. Using ½ cup measuring cup scoop out mix and combine and form to make patty. Set aside all patties. Preheat skillet over medium heat and add canola oil. Once pan is hot add crab cake patty and cook 4-5 minutes each side until golden brown and warmed through. Serve on your favorite whole grain bun, lettuce wrap or make smaller patties and serve as an appetizer. -Enjoy!

Honey Dew Whole Grain Chicken Pita

1 lime juiced and zested
3-4 cooked 6-ounce chicken breasts cubed
½ honey dew cleaned and diced small
2 celery stalks washed and thinly sliced or minced
2 scallions chopped
1-tblsp. Fresh chopped mint
1 seedless cucumber peeled and diced
¼ cup mayonnaise
1 bunch watercress washed and chopped
4 whole-wheat pitas

Mix all ingredients except watercress and pita in large mixing bowl and toss to incorporate flavor well. Set in fridge to cool before serving, this can be made a day ahead of time. Slice pitas open and add chicken mixture in with small handful of watercress. Serve and Enjoy!

Chicken BLT (Bacon, Lettuce and Tart Cherries)

8 slices thick cooked bacon (or pancetta works great)
4-4oz. boneless skinless chicken breasts pounded and cooked
Leaf lettuce or Romaine
½ cup tart cherries pitted and chopped
½ cup orange juice
1-tblsp. Fresh cilantro
4 Ciabatta buns or your favorite whole grain bun will do

Cook bacon in oven at 425 until crisp and cooked through. Remove and cool to room temp on paper towels. Heat canola oil in skillet and cook chicken 4-6 minutes a side until cooked through and golden brown. Remove from heat and cool to room temp. In small saucepan heat cherries and orange juice and cilantro over high heat for 3 minutes stirring. Reduce heat to medium and cook for 10 minutes until it reduces by half and thickens. Remove from heat and set aside to cool to room temp. Arrange your sandwich by placing 2 pieces bacon, leaf lettuce, chicken on bun then drizzling cherry compote over the top and serve. –Enjoy!

Lemon and Herb Grilled Trout Sandwich

1 pound ruby or rainbow trout filets, deboned and cleaned
4 Ciabatta buns or your favorite whole grain bun
1 lemon zested and juiced
1 lime zested and juiced
1-tblsp. Fresh chopped basil
1-tblsp. Fresh thyme
1-tblsp Fresh tarragon
2-tblsp Canola oil

Combine juice and zest of lemon and lime in bowl and add herbs. Mix well and set aside. Heat oil in skillet and when hot add trout to skillet. Start basting the trout with herb mixture. Baste the fish while cooking 3-4 minutes aside until the fish is cooked through and flaky. Remove from heat and cool to room temp. Place fish on your bun of choice. -Enjoy!
- You can add watercress or romaine to this sandwich and drizzle with a bit of olive oil for nice texture and flavor.

Facial Friendly Breakfast Pita

2 pits cut in half
3 organic eggs
1 medium potato, cleaned peeled and diced small
1-tblsp. Fresh cilantro chopped
1-tblsp. Fresh chopped garlic 2 shallots diced and minced
2-tblsp. Canola oil

Heat oil in skillet on medium/high heat and place potatoes in. Sauté for 5-7 minutes stirring occasionally, add in onion and garlic. Cook for another 2 minutes reducing heat to medium. Beat eggs in bowl and add to skillet and stir 45 seconds, add herbs last and remove from heat. Heat pita in oven or microwave for 30 seconds and scoop egg mixture into pita and serve. Let this cool to room temp before you eat. -Enjoy!

Entrees & Pasta's

Walnut and Rosemary Crusted Baked Cod

1/3-cup walnuts (use almond or pecan if allergic)
1/3-cup fresh whole grain bread crumbs
2-tblsp. Fresh chopped rosemary (I blend mine in blender or food processor for 20 seconds)
1-tblsp. Fresh thyme pulled from stem
2-tblsp. Canola oil
2 egg whites
1 lemon juiced and zested
4-4oz. cod filets cleaned

Preheat oven to 400 degrees. In small bowl mix together breadcrumbs, walnuts, lemon zest, fresh thyme and rosemary and toss to mix evenly. In separate bowl beat 2 egg whites and lemon juice with fork. Heat oil in skillet to medium heat. Dredge filets of cod into egg mixture and then dip into breadcrumb mix and coat evenly on all sides. Sear fish in skillet for 3-4 minutes until golden brown on all sides. Remove from heat and place fish on baking sheet or leave in skillet and add to oven and finish baking for 8-10 minutes. Remove fish from oven and place on serving dish and let sit to cool to room temp. Serve dish with your favorite side and Enjoy!

- Garnish with fresh thyme and drizzle with olive oil for a nice finish.

Whole Grain Ziti Finished with Lemon and Brussels sprouts

¾ lb. Brussels sprouts
1 lemon juiced and zested
2 shallots sliced and minced

3 cloves garlic chopped
2-tblsp. Fresh chopped basil
1-tblsp. Fresh chopped oregano
1 leek (white parts only sliced thinly)
1 cup white wine of choice (dry preferably)
1 lb. Whole grain ziti
3-tblsp. Canola oil

Clean and trim Brussels sprouts by removing outer dark leaf and cut in half or quarter each sprout. Cut thin slices form white part off leek and add to mixing bowl with sprouts. Toss herbs into bowl with t-tblsp. Canola oil and lemon juice and zest from lemon. Set aside in fridge to chill while you cook the pasta. Bring together salted water in large stockpot to boil and cook ziti for 8-10 minutes until you find it al dente (to the tooth). Remove and strain pasta, do not rinse and let cool to room temperature. Heat skillet with 1-tblsp. Canola oil and bring to medium heat. Add Brussels sprouts mixture to skillet and white wine and cook stirring the sprouts for 4-6 minutes. Reduce heat to low and toss in noodles a handful at a time. Mix well and remove from heat after 2 minutes and plate in serving dishes or bowls. Garnish with additional lemon juice if desired and some fresh chopped basil. –Enjoy!
-   Some fresh Parmesan cheese will do this dish great to finish, but keep in mind this has high levels of histamine and will aggravate your rosacea symptoms.

Pomegranate Baked Salmon with Tart Cherry Saffron Rice

4 salmon filets 6-8oz. cleaned
¼ cup orange juice
¼ cup pomegranate juice

For the rice:
3-cups vegetable stock
2-cups instant whole grain rice
1 pinch saffron threads
5-tblsp. Fresh-pitted cherries
1-tblsp fresh chopped mint
Sea salt and olive oil for garnish

Bring orange juice and pomegranate juice to boil in saucepot and let cook 10-12 minutes until reduces by half and becomes thick. Remove from heat and set aside to cool. Preheat oven to 400 degrees. For the rice bring stock, rice, and saffron to a boil and reduce heat to medium stirring frequently for 6-8 minutes. Add in fresh cherries, mint, and stir to mix. Remove from heat and set aside to cool. Place salmon filets in baking dish and spoon ½ pomegranate sauce over fish and place in oven for 5-6 minutes. Remove from oven and spoon rest of sauce (reserving about 1-tblsp.) over fish and bake an additional 6-8 minutes. Remove fish from oven and let cool to room temp. Assemble your fish on plates over bed of rice and drizzle any remaining sauce over filets and serve. -Enjoy!

Seared Chicken with Fresh Blackberry Compote

4 chicken breasts (boneless and skinned)
2-tblsp. Canola oil
½ cup fresh blackberries
1-tblsp. Fresh chopped mint
¼ cup orange juice
1 lemon juiced and zested
2-tblsp. Cognac

In a small saucepan bring lemon juice, orange juice, and blackberries to boil and reduce to medium heat. Cook for additional 6-8 minutes until reduces by half and add in fresh mint and zest form lemon. Remove from heat and set aside to cool at room temp. In a skillet heat canola oil in pan to medium heat and add chicken. Sear and cook 6-8 minutes aside until chicken is cooked through and tender. Remove from heat and set aside. Place chicken on serving dish and scoop blackberry compote over chicken and server with your favorite side. –Enjoy!

Cherry, Kale, and Pancetta Stuffed Chicken

4 chicken breasts boneless, skinned
5 slices pancetta cooked (or thick cut bacon will work)
½ bunch washed and chopped kale
3 cloves garlic chopped and minced
2 shallots minced (or ¼ small yellow onion)
½ cup washed, pitted and chopped cherries

3-tblsp. Canola oil
1-tblsp. Fresh thyme

Preheat oven to 375 degrees. Take and pound out your chicken so that the lobes are even with rest of breast. This prevents drying out the chicken. In a skillet heat oil to medium heat and add garlic, shallots, pancetta, and cherries. Mix this for about 3-4 minutes. Add kale and thyme and toss to mix well for another 2 minutes until kale starts to break down. Remove from heat and set aside to cool to room temp. While this cools take chicken and cut slit in lobe that you pounded out earlier with paring knife about ½ inch deep and wide, or cut chicken breasts in half if this is easier and you can spread the mixture on it that way (like making a sandwich). Now take the cherry/kale mixture and stuff it into the whole you cut in the chicken with small spoon or use your fingers and stuff it in there. Once this tedious step is done heat skillet with oil and sear chicken in skillet for 4-6 minutes a side until golden brown and has a nice sear. Remove from heat and place skillet in oven or use baking dish and bake chicken for 6-8 minutes more. Remove form oven and set aside to cool at room temp. Plate this on serving dishes with your favorite side. – Enjoy!

Crispy Tofu Finished with Mixed Vegetable and Mushroom Medley

1 pound extra firm, pressed tofu, (I press between plates for 3-5 minutes)
2-tblsp. Canola oil
½ lb. fresh shitake mushrooms sliced
¼ lb. fresh crimini mushrooms sliced
½ head broccoli cleaned and chopped
¼ lb. green beans cleaned and chopped
2-tblsp. Sesame oil
3-tblsp. Sesame seeds, roasted for 2 minutes in oven
½ bunch scallions washed and chopped
2 shallots sliced and minced
1 clove garlic minced
2-tblsp fresh chopped cilantro

Slice the tofu in ½ inch squares and ½ inch thick after pressing. Set aside.

Heat 1-tblsp. Canola oil in skillet over medium heat and sear tofu in oil 3-5 minutes a side until golden brown. Cook this in small batches until it is all crispy and then place on paper plate lined with paper towel to dry out. In the same skillet add the remaining oil, garlic, scallions, green beans and broccoli. Cook stirring for 3 minutes over medium heat. Add mushrooms, sesame seeds, and sesame oil and cook another 2 minutes stirring. Remove from heat and toss in cilantro and mix to incorporate. Remove from heat and let cool to room temp. Plate with tofu on serving dish and top with mushroom/vegetable medley. -Enjoy!

Pappardelle with Chicken Sugo and Walnuts

1-lb. fresh or dried Pappardelle
6 cloves garlic smashed and minced
4-tblsp. Canola oil
½ cup blanched walnuts (hazelnut or pecan will work if you are allergic to walnut)
2-lb. boneless skinless chicken breasts
5 shallots chopped and minced
2 cups white wine (I use a pinot) plus 1 cup to use at end
1 ½-cups Almond milk
1 ½-cups vegetable broth
6 sprigs fresh Thyme chopped
6 sprigs fresh Oregano chopped
2-tbslp. Fresh chopped basil
1-tblsp. Organic butter

Preheat oven to 350 degrees. Place chicken breasts in baking dish and cook for 25 minutes until cooked through and remove to cool to room temp. Cut chicken into ½ inch cubes and set aside. Place walnuts on baking dish and cook 8-10 minutes, remove from oven and set aside to cool. Once cool chop walnuts roughly and set aside. Heat large stockpot with canola oil to medium heat, add shallots and garlic and stir. Cook about 4-6 minutes then add the wine and scrape the pot with wooden spoon and reduce heat after 5 minutes to simmer. Add chicken, vegetable broth, and milk to pot. Bring to a boil for 10 minutes. Reduce heat to simmer and add in fresh herbs. Cook this on stove at low simmer for 1-½ hours stirring frequently. Add in butter at lest step and the additional 1 cup white wine. Cook an additional 30 minutes at low simmer while stirring frequently. Meanwhile, cook your pasta in stockpot in salted water, stirring occasionally for 6-8 minutes. Once pasta is al dente remove and strain from water. Remove chicken sugo from stove and let cool to room temp. Plate your pasta on serving dishes and scoop chicken sugo over pasta. Sprinkle chopped walnuts over finished pasta and serve. -Enjoy!

-   This can be garnished with fresh Parmesan cheese or Romano. However cheese is full of histamine and can aggravate our rosacea. The chicken sugo can be made up to 5 days ahead and stored in fridge, this sauce builds better flavor the following days after it is cooked. You can also freeze the leftover sauce for up to 2 months.

Pan Seared Flounder Piccata

4 skinless flounder filets
1-tblsp. Flax seed
2-tblsp. Canola oil
2 shallots chopped and minced
1 lemon juiced and zested
1 cup white wine (dry)
1-tblsp. Organic butter
½ cup capers

Wash filets and pat dry. Put flaxseed in small bowl and coat your flounder in flaxseed to coat evenly. Set aside to cook. Place oil in skillet and heat to medium. Cook flounder filets in skillet 4-6 minutes a side until cooked through and golden brown. Remove from skillet and set on serving dish to cool. Take same skillet and replace on heat, add shallot, wine, lemon juice, zest, and capers and bring to small boil. Reduce heat after 2 minutes and add in butter stir. Cook for another 1 minute until sauce becomes thick and remove from heat. Drizzle sauce over your flounder filets and serve with your favorite side. –Enjoy!

Incredible Turkey Meatloaf Finished with Pomegranate and Blueberry

1-tblsp. Canola oil
2 cloves garlic smashed and minced

½ cup vegetable broth or stock
2-lbs. Ground turkey
1-cup fresh whole grain breadcrumbs (I rip apart a few pieces of whole grain bread into fine pieces)
2 large organic eggs beaten
2-tblsp. Fresh chopped thyme
1-tblsp. Fresh chopped cilantro
2 shallots minced or ¼ small yellow onion chopped
1-cup pomegranate juice
½ cup blueberries

Preheat oven to 375 degrees. Combine all ingredients except oil, pomegranate juice, and blueberries in large mixing bowl and fold into each well to incorporate the flavors. Oil your loaf pan or baking dish with canola oil and scoop turkey mixture into pan evenly with spatula and flatten firmly. Set aside. In a small saucepot bring pomegranate Juice and blueberries to boil and reduce heat to low after 5 minutes. Once this has begun to thicken and reduce by half remove from heat and set aside to cool. Spoon blueberry mix (reserving about 3-tblsp.) over turkey loaf to coat evenly and place in oven to bake for 55-65 minutes or until thermometer reaches an internal temp of 170 degrees. Remove from oven and cool to room temp. Spoon the last of the blueberry sauce over turkey loaf, cut and serve. -Enjoy!

Beautiful Flaxseed Crusted Ahi Tuna Steak

2-4 6ounce Fresh Ahi Tuna Steaks from market
2-tblsp. Flaxseed
1-tblsp. Fresh chopped mint
1 lemon juiced and zested
1 lime juice and zested
2-tblsp. Canola oil
¼ cup white wine (dry)

Combine the flaxseed, mint, lemon and lime zest in small mixing bowl and combine to incorporate flavors. Dredge your ahi tuna steaks in mixture to coat evenly. Set aside. Heat canola oil in skillet to medium/high heat and cook your tuna for 45 seconds a side to sear and reduce heat to medium. Add wine and cook your tuna for 1 minute a side and flip and cook other side for 1 minute. Remove from heat and set aside to cool. Take your tuna out after cooled and cut into ½ strips with sharp knife against the grain diagonally. Serve this dish over a bed of fresh watercress or arugula with a drizzle of olive oil for best results. –Enjoy!

Desserts and Healthy Snacks

Coconut and Sesame Seed Walnut Bars

1 ½ cups white and black sesame seeds
2-tblsp. Flaxseed
1 cup shredded coconut (sweetened)
½ cup chopped walnuts (hazelnut or pecan will work if your allergic)
¼ cup raw organic honey
3-tblsp. Peanut butter (creamy)
1-tblsp. Fresh chopped mint
2-tblsp. Canola oil

Preheat oven to 350 degrees. In a mixing bowl add sesame seeds, flaxseed, coconut, and honey and blend well. Fold in walnuts, oil, and mint and blend to incorporate. Mix in peanut butter last and blend well. Line a baking dish with parchment paper and lightly grease with canola oil. Take and scoop mixture into oil greased baking dish and press into pan to make firm. Bake this for 22-25 minutes. Remove from oven and let cool. Lift to remove this from pan carefully and set aside to cool to room temp. Cut into your desired squares or use cookie cutters and make shapes. Serve and Enjoy!
- The leftovers can be stored in airtight container for up to 5 days.

Carrot Cake with Coconut Cream Cheese

Makes a 8-9 inch two layer cake

1-cup whole-wheat pastry flour
1-cup all purpose flour
1-tblsp. Baking soda
1-cup light brown sugar
1-cup granulated sugar

1-¼ cups canola oil
1 cup chopped walnuts (almond or pecan if allergic)
5 large organic eggs
4 cups finely grated peeled carrots (about 8 carrots)
1-tsp. ground nutmeg

Preheat oven to 350 degrees. Grease and line your pans of choice (circle or square 8 inch or 9inch).

In a medium bowl, combine you dry ingredients and mix well. In a separate bowl mix together sugar and oil until it is blended in well. Beat in eggs one at a time. Add the flour mixture and fold in with spatula a little at a time. Add the carrots and walnuts in last. Divide the batter into your prepared pans. Bake the cakes for 45-55 minutes. Or until you stick with clean knife and it comes out clean. Remove and let cool to room temp before removing from cake pans.

For the cream cheese:
2 package tofu cream cheese
½ cup shredded unsweetened coconut
1-tblsp. Apple cider vinegar
2-tblsp. Almond milk
½ cup grated carrot
1-cup sugar

Combine all ingredients in mixing bowl with spatula and fold in well to incorporate. Spread your frosting on your cake and assemble your cake. Cut, serve and enjoy!

Pomegranate and Cherry Sorbet

2 ½-cups pomegranate juice
1-cup fresh or frozen chopped cherries (blended in blender until smooth)
½ cup sugar
½ cup honey
1-tblsp. Fresh chopped mint
I lime juiced and zested
½ cup filtered water

Combine limejuice, zest and pomegranate juice and cherries in large bowl. Add ½ cup filtered water, sugar, honey and mint to incorporate. Pour this mixture and process this in an ice cream machine for 30-40 minutes or until it begins to firm up. Remove and transfer to airtight container to store over night and let it settle and firm up. Let sit at least 3-hours in freezer before serving. When ready to serve, scoop some sorbet into glasses or serving bowls and garnish with fresh chopped mint. –Enjoy!
-Sprinkle toasted pistachio or walnuts over top for added texture and great flavor. This can store in freezer for up to 3 weeks.

<u>Delicious Matcha Green Tea Doughnuts</u>
Makes 8

¼ cup granulated sugar
2-tsp. baking powder
2 cups cake flour plus extra for flouring prep surface
1 large organic egg
½ cup almond milk or silk vanilla soy
2-tblsp. Butter (melted)
3-5 cups canola oil for frying

Start by whisking sugar, baking powder and flour in a mixing bowl. Add melted butter and egg and fold to incorporate with spatula. Continue to fold until dough forms and becomes firm. Turn out onto a floured work surface or cutting board. Knead this dough a few times over and over but not too much, you don't want to over work the dough. Knead for about 1 minute. Roll out your dough to ½ inch thick, use flour and coat if start to sticks. Punch out as many circled doughnuts as you can with your 3-¼ inch cutter. Then set aside. Now use your 1-¼ inch cutter and punch out centers for each round. Reserve these and either re-roll and make more or use for making doughnut holes the kids will be sure to enjoy. Bring oil up to temperature in medium sized saucepan. Use your thermometer to determine when he oil is hot enough for frying these. You want your oil at least 325 degrees or at the most 350 degrees. Cook your doughnuts dropping in one at a time, wait 45 seconds and drop in another, don't overcrowd the pot or they will stick. Cook for about 3-4 minutes until golden brown and remove with slotted spoon and set aside to cool on paper towel lined plates to dry. Let cool but not completely before you toss to coat in your topping of choice.

For the toppings:

<u>Green Tea Matcha Sugar Coating</u>

Whisk together ½ cup granulated sugar with 1-tblsp. Green tea matcha with fork in small bowl or whisk until incorporated smoothly. Coat in your doughnuts and Enjoy!

<u>Green Tea Matcha Glaze</u>

In a shallow bowl whisk 1 large organic egg with 1-½ cups of powdered sugar. Mix thoroughly. Add in 1-tblsp. Matcha powder and 1 tablespoon Filtered water and incorporate with fork or whisk until smooth. Coat on top of your doughnut of choice with a small spoon and Enjoy!

Fresh Berries and Bread Pudding

4 large organic eggs
1 ½ cups organic sugar
1 ½ cups fresh or frozen blueberries
1 ½ cups fresh or frozen pitted cherries
1 whole grain loaf of bread cut into ½ inch cubes (or tear with fingers to create pieces)
4 cups almond milk or silk vanilla soy
2-tblsp. Fresh chopped mint
1 cup chopped walnuts (optional)
2-tblsp. Canola oil for greasing

Preheat oven to 350 degrees. In a small saucepan heat almond milk and sugar to a boil and reduce heat. Cook 1 minute and remove from heat. In large mixing bowl combine berries, bread, mint, eggs and walnuts (optional) and mix thoroughly. Add in milk mixture and fold to incorporate. Grease a 13x9-baking dish with canola oil and pour bread mixture into pan. Bake uncovered for 45-55 minutes or until knife inserted comes out clean. Remove from oven and let cool to room temp. Cut squares out of pan and serve with your favorite ice cream or alone. This can be kept in fridge in airtight container for up to 5 days. –Enjoy!

Whole Wheat Blueberry and Peach Cobbler

1-cup whole-wheat pastry flour or whole-wheat flour
1 cup almond milk or silk vanilla soy
½ cup organic sugar
3-tblsp. Canola oil
3-tblsp. Unsalted organic butter
4 cups peaches fresh or frozen and pitted and chopped
3 cups fresh or frozen blueberries

Preheat oven to 350 degrees. In cast-iron skillet heat butter and oil on low heat until it becomes melted. About 3 minutes. Remove from heat and in large mixing bowl combine wheat flour, baking powder and sugar and mix to combine. Add in your butter, and milk and stir in to incorporate. Pour the batter into the skillet and spoon berries and peaches over batter evenly. Place skillet in oven and bake for 55-65 minutes. Remove from oven and let cool to room temp. Cut your desired piece, serve and Enjoy!
- This can also be made in a glass baking dish 8x8 or 9x13. And a scoop of organic vanilla ice cream on top with some fresh mint will complete this nicely.

Berries & Grain Snack Bars

2-cups whole-wheat pastry flour or whole-wheat flour
1 ½ cups plain oats (old-fashioned)
1 cup chopped walnuts (pecans or almond will work to if allergic)
2-tblsp. Flaxseed (optional)
2-tsp. baking soda
1-tsp. baking powder
1-cup melted butter (organic)
3 large organic eggs
¼ cup honey
¼ cup shredded coconut
2 ½ cups fresh pitted and chopped cherries
½ cup fresh chopped blueberries
1-tblsp. Fresh chopped mint

Preheat oven to 350 degrees. In a large bowl combine the flour, walnuts, flaxseed, baking soda and powder, oats and combine to mix well. In a smaller bowl mix together your honey, butter, eggs and coconut. Mix well to combine the flavors. Stir this egg mix into oat mixture and fold in to incorporate well. Remove about 1 cup to small bowl for later use. Grease a baking dish 13x9 with canola oil and press oat mix into pan firmly, spreading evenly. Top with your fresh berries and spread evenly. Now toss remaining mixture form small bowl over the top evenly and spread out. Bake this for 27-32 minutes or until golden brown on top. Remove from oven and let cool to room temp. Cut into your desired size bars, serve and Enjoy!

- You can also use frozen berries with this and substitute your berries with say blackberries or even strawberries. Pack rest of bars in airtight container and store for up to 1 week.

__Whole Wheat Peaches and Apple Crisp__

1-cup whole-wheat pastry flour or whole-wheat flour
½ cup organic sugar
6-tblsp. Coconut oil
½ cup chopped walnuts (pecans or almonds if allergic)
5 cups peeled and diced apples
1 ½ cups frozen or fresh chopped peaches (skinned)
1-tsp cinnamon
1/3-cup apple jam or jelly
2-tblsp. Canola oil

Preheat oven to 350 degrees. Grease a skillet or baking dish 9x13 or 8x8 with canola oil. Prepare the filling by mixing in a large bowl the apples, peaches, cinnamon, and jam or jelly. Set aside. In separate bowl mix together the coconut oil, walnuts, sugar and flour. Combine thoroughly and set aside. Scoop the filling mixture into you baking dish of choice and spread evenly around and press lightly into pan.
Sprinkle the topping over the top spreading evenly to coat entire thing. Place in oven and bake for 35-45 minutes or until bubbly and golden brown on top. Remove from oven and let cool to room temp. Cut your desired slice, serve and Enjoy!

- This is great with some organic vanilla or coconut ice cream on top.

Sweet Cherry Pie Cookies

4-tblsp. Coconut oil
2-cups whole-wheat pastry flour
½ cup organic sugar
3-tblsp. Organic butter softened
1-cup fresh or frozen pitted chopped tart cherries
1-tblsp. Canola oil
1-tsp. fresh chopped mint (optional)

Preheat oven to 325 degrees. Mix coconut oil, and butter in mixing bowl and whisk until incorporated. Add flour, sugar and mix well. Combine the butter mix into bowl and mix together to fold in the flavors and ingredients until soft dough is formed. In separate bowl mix mint with cherries set aside. Roll the dough into 1-½ inch balls. Lightly grease a baking sheet with canola oil. Place cookies on sheet 1 inch apart and press into each with thumb to make a well on top of each cookie. Spoon cherry mixture on to well of each cookie. Bake your cookies for 13-15 minutes. Remove from oven and let cool to room temp. Serve and Enjoy!

Mixed Berry Granola and Flaxseed Parfait

¼ cup fresh raspberries
¼ cup fresh blueberries
¼ cup fresh chopped strawberries
5-tblsp. Filtered water
¼ cup plain granola (with nuts optional)
2-tblsp. Flaxseed
1-½ cups dairy free plain yogurt (flavored is fine to like vanilla)
2-tblsp. Honey

Bring strawberries and raspberries with water to low boil, add honey and reduce while mashing berries with slotted spoon or whisk. Remove from heat and let cool to room temp. While that is cooling take the serving dish or cup

of choice and layer the granola, yogurt, flaxseeds then blueberries. Once the raspberry mixture is cooled down pour over the blueberry yogurt mixture. Repeat with granola, flax, and yogurt mix. Serve and Enjoy!
-   Garnish with fresh chopped mint